Mediterranean Diet Cookbook Quick and Easy

For Optimum Body Health with Mediterranean Diet and Lifestyle. Healthy Cooking with Easy Recipes

Kelly R. Boyd

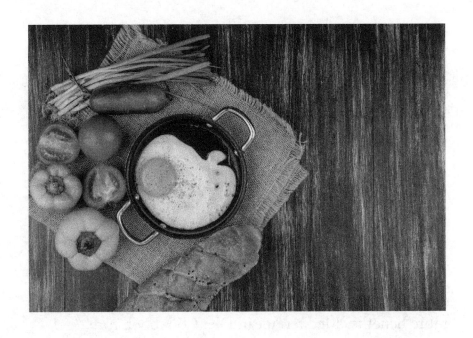

The Mediterranean Diet Cookbook for Beginners are two of the most consistently recommended for optimal health and well-being, so why not combine them and get even more benefits? Mediterranean Diet Cookbook for Beginners offers simple recipes that adhere to both diets, helping you lower your blood pressure and maintain good health—without sacrificing flavor or convenience.

Table Of Contents

Artichoke and Olive Pita Flatbread

Preparation Time : 5 minutes

Cooking Time : 10 minutes

Servings : 4

Difficulty Level : Easy

Ingredients:

2 whole wheat pitas

2 tablespoons olive oil, divided

2 garlic cloves, minced

¼ teaspoon salt

½ cup canned artichoke hearts, sliced

¼ cup Kalamata olives

¼ cup shredded Parmesan

¼ cup crumbled feta

Chopped fresh parsley, for garnish (optional)

Directions:

1. Preheat the air fryer to 380°F. Brush each pita with 1 tablespoon olive oil, then sprinkle the

minced garlic and salt over the top.

2. Distribute the artichoke hearts, olives, and cheeses evenly between the two pitas, and place both

into the air fryer to bake for 10 minutes. Remove the pitas and cut them into 4 pieces each

before serving. Sprinkle parsley over the top, if desired.

Nutrition (for 100g): 243 Calories 15g Fat 10g Carbohydrates 7g Protein 644mg Sodium

Mini Crab Cakes

Preparation Time : 10 minutes

Cooking Time : 10 minutes

Servings : 6

Difficulty Level : Average

Ingredients:

8 ounces lump crab meat

2 tablespoons diced red bell pepper

1 scallion, white parts and green parts, diced

1 garlic clove, minced

1 tablespoon capers, minced

1 tablespoon nonfat plain Greek yogurt

1 egg, beaten

¼ cup whole wheat bread crumbs

¼ teaspoon salt

1 tablespoon olive oil

1 lemon, cut into wedges

Directions:

1. Preheat the air fryer to 360°F. In a medium bowl, mix the crab, bell pepper, scallion, garlic, and

capers until combined. Add the yogurt and egg. Stir until incorporated. Mix in the bread crumbs and salt.

2. Portion this mixture into 6 equal parts and pat out into patties. Place the crab cakes inside the

air fryer basket on single layer, separately. Grease the tops of each patty with a bit of olive oil.

Bake for 10 minutes.

3. Remove the crab cakes from the air fryer and serve with lemon wedges on the side.

Nutrition (for 100g): 87 Calories 4g Fat 6g Carbohydrates 9g Protein 574mg Sodium

Zucchini Feta Roulades

Preparation Time : 10 minutes

Cooking Time : 10 minutes

Servings : 6

Difficulty Level : Average

Ingredients:

½ cup feta

1 garlic clove, minced

2 tablespoons fresh basil, minced

1 tablespoon capers, minced

1/8 teaspoon salt

1/8 teaspoon red pepper flakes

1 tablespoon lemon juice

2 medium zucchinis

12 toothpicks

Directions:

1. Preheat the air fryer to 360°F. (If using a grill attachment, make sure it is inside the air fryer

during preheating.) In a small bowl, mix the feta, garlic, basil, capers, salt, red pepper flakes,

and lemon juice.

2. Slice the zucchini into 1/8-inch strips lengthwise. (Each zucchini should yield around 6 strips.)

Spread 1 tablespoon of the cheese filling onto each slice of zucchini, then roll it up and locked it with a toothpick through the middle.

3. Place the zucchini roulades into the air fryer basket in a one layer, individually. Bake or grill in

the air fryer for 10 minutes. Remove the zucchini roulades from the air fryer and gently remove

the toothpicks before serving.

Nutrition (for 100g): 46 Calories 3g Fat 6g Carbohydrates 3g Protein 710mg Sodium

Garlic-Roasted Tomatoes and Olives

Preparation Time : 5 minutes

Cooking Time : 20 minutes

Servings : 6

Difficulty Level : EasyIngredients:

2 cups cherry tomatoes

4 garlic cloves, roughly chopped

½ red onion, roughly chopped

1 cup black olives

1 cup green olives

1 tablespoon fresh basil, minced

1 tablespoon fresh oregano, minced

2 tablespoons olive oil

¼ to ½ teaspoon salt

Directions:

1. Preheat the air fryer to 380°F. In a large bowl, incorporate all of the ingredients and toss

together so that the tomatoes and olives are coated well with the olive oil and herbs.

2. Pour the mixture into the air fryer basket, and roast for 10 minutes. Stir the mixture well, then

continue roasting for an additional 10 minutes. Remove from the air fryer, transfer to a serving

bowl, and enjoy.

Nutrition (for 100g): 109 Calories 10g Fat 5g Carbohydrates 1g Protein 647mg Sodium

Goat Cheese and Garlic Crostini

Preparation Time : 3 minutes

Cooking Time : 5 minutes

Servings : 4

Difficulty Level : Average

Ingredients:

1 whole wheat baguette

¼ cup olive oil

2 garlic cloves, minced

4 ounces goat cheese

2 tablespoons fresh basil, minced

Directions:

1. Preheat the air fryer to 380°F. Cut the baguette into ½-inch-thick slices. In a small bowl,

incorporate together the olive oil and garlic, then brush it over one side of each slice of bread.

2. Place the olive-oil-coated bread in a single layer in the air fryer basket and bake for 5 minutes. In

the meantime, combine together the goat cheese and basil. Remove the toast from the air fryer,

then spread a thin layer of the goat cheese mixture over on each piece and serve.

Nutrition (for 100g): 365 Calories 21g Fat 10g Carbohydrates 12g Protein 804mg Sodium

Rosemary-Roasted Red Potatoes

Preparation Time : 5 minutes

Cooking Time : 20 minutes

Servings : 6

Difficulty Level : Easy

Ingredients:

1-pound red potatoes, quartered

¼ cup olive oil

½ teaspoon kosher salt

¼ teaspoon black pepper

1 garlic clove, minced

4 rosemary sprigs

Directions:

1. Preheat the air fryer to 360°F.

2. In a large bowl, toss in the potatoes with the olive oil, salt, pepper, and garlic until well coated.

Fill the air fryer basket with potatoes and top with the sprigs of rosemary.

3. Roast for 10 minutes, then stir or toss the potatoes and roast for 10 minutes more. Remove the

rosemary sprigs and serve the potatoes. Season well.Nutrition (for 100g): 133 Calories 9g Fat 5g Carbohydrates 1g Protein 617mg Sodium

Avocado Egg Scramble

Preparation Time : 8 minutes

Cooking Time : 15 minutes

Servings : 4

Difficulty Level : Average

Ingredients:

4 eggs, beaten

1 white onion, diced

1 tablespoon avocado oil

1 avocado, finely chopped

½ teaspoon chili flakes

1 oz Cheddar cheese, shredded

½ teaspoon salt

1 tablespoon fresh parsley

Directions:

4. Pour avocado oil in the skillet and bring it to boil. Then add diced onion and roast it until it is

light brown. Meanwhile, mix up together chili flakes, beaten eggs, and salt.

5. Fill the egg mixture over the cooked onion and cook the mixture for 1 minute over the medium

heat. After this, scramble the eggs well with the help of the fork or spatula. Cook the eggs until

they are solid but soft.

6. After this, add chopped avocado and shredded cheese. Stir the scramble well and transfer in the

serving plates. Sprinkle the meal with fresh parsley.

Nutrition (for 100g): 236 Calories 20g Fat 4g Carbohydrates 6g Protein 804mg Sodium

Morning Tostadas

Preparation Time : 15 minutes

Cooking Time : 6 minutes

Servings : 6

Difficulty Level : Difficult

Ingredients :

½ white onion, diced

1 tomato, chopped

1 cucumber, chopped

1 tablespoon fresh cilantro, chopped

½ jalapeno pepper, chopped

1 tablespoon lime juice

6 corn tortillas

1 tablespoon canola oil

2 oz Cheddar cheese, shredded

½ cup white beans, canned, drained

6 eggs

½ teaspoon butter

½ teaspoon Sea salt

Directions:

1. Make Pico de Galo: in the salad bowl combine together diced white onion, tomato, cucumber,

fresh cilantro, and jalapeno pepper. Then add lime juice and a ½ tablespoon of canola oil. Mix up

the mixture well. Pico de Galo is cooked. After this, preheat the oven to 390F. Line the tray with

baking paper. Arrange the corn tortillas on the baking paper and brush with remaining canola oil

from both sides. Bake the tortillas until they start to be crunchy. Chill the cooked crunchy

tortillas well. Meanwhile, toss the butter in the skillet.

2. Crack the eggs in the melted butter and sprinkle them with sea salt. Fry the eggs until the egg

whites become white (cooked). Approximately for 3-5 minutes over the medium heat. After this, mash the beans until you get puree texture. Spread the bean puree on the corn tortillas. Add

fried eggs. Then top the eggs with Pico de Galo and shredded Cheddar cheese.

Nutrition (for 100g): 246 Calories 11g Fat 7g Carbohydrates 7g Protein 593mg Sodium

Parmesan Omelet

Preparation Time : 5 minutes

Cooking Time : 10 minutes

Servings : 2

Difficulty Level : Easy

Ingredients:

1 tablespoon cream cheese

2 eggs, beaten

¼ teaspoon paprika

½ teaspoon dried oregano

¼ teaspoon dried dill

1 oz Parmesan, grated

1 teaspoon coconut oil

Directions:

1. Mix up together cream cheese with eggs, dried oregano, and dill. Pour coconut oil in the skillet

and heat it up until it will coat all the skillet. Then fill the skillet with the egg mixture and flatten

it. Add grated Parmesan and close the lid. Cook omelet for 10 minutes over the low heat. Then

transfer the cooked omelet in the serving plate and sprinkle with paprika.

Nutrition (for 100g): 148 Calories 5g Fat 3g Carbohydrates 6g Protein 741mg Sodium

Watermelon Pizza

Preparation Time : 10 minutes

Cooking Time : 0 minutes

Servings : 2

Difficulty Level : Easy

Ingredients:

9 oz watermelon slice

1 tablespoon Pomegranate sauce

2 oz Feta cheese, crumbled

1 tablespoon fresh cilantro, chopped

Directions:

1. Place the watermelon slice in the plate and sprinkle with crumbled Feta cheese. Add fresh

cilantro. After this, sprinkle the pizza with Pomegranate juice generously. Cut the pizza into the

servings.

Nutrition (for 100g): 143 Calories 2g Fat 6g Carbohydrates 1g Protein 811mg Sodium

Savory Muffins

Preparation Time : 10 minutes

Cooking Time : 15 minutes

Servings : 4

Difficulty Level : Average

Ingredients:

3 oz ham, chopped

4 eggs, beaten

2 tablespoons coconut flour

½ teaspoon dried oregano

¼ teaspoon dried cilantro

Cooking spray

Directions:

1. Spray the muffin's molds with cooking spray from inside. In the bowl mix up together beaten

eggs, coconut flour, dried oregano, cilantro, and ham. When the liquid is homogenous, pour it in

the prepared muffin molds.

2. Bake the muffins for 15 minutes at 360F. Chill the cooked meal well and only after this remove

from the molds.

Nutrition (for 100g): 128 Calories 2g Fat 9g Carbohydrates 1g Protein 882mg Sodium

Morning Pizza with Sprouts

Preparation Time : 15 minutes

Cooking Time : 20 minutes

Servings : 6

Difficulty Level : Average

Ingredients :

½ cup wheat flour, whole grain

2 tablespoons butter, softened

¼ teaspoon baking powder

¾ teaspoon salt

5 oz chicken fillet, boiled

2 oz Cheddar cheese, shredded

1 teaspoon tomato sauce

1 oz bean sprouts

Directions :

1. Make the pizza crust: mix up together wheat flour, butter, baking powder, and salt. Knead the

soft and non-sticky dough. Add more wheat flour if needed. Leave the dough for 10 minutes to

chill. Then place the dough on the baking paper. Cover it with the second baking paper sheet.

2. Roll up the dough with the help of the rolling pin to get the round pizza crust. After this, remove

the upper baking paper sheet. Transfer the pizza crust in the tray.

3. Spread the crust with tomato sauce. Then shred the chicken fillet and arrange it over the pizza

crust. Add shredded Cheddar cheese. Bake pizza for 20 minutes at 355F. Then top the cooked

pizza with bean sprouts and slice into the servings.

Nutrition (for 100g): 157 Calories 8g Fat 3g Carbohydrates 5g Protein 753mg Sodium

Banana Quinoa

Preparation Time : 10 minutes

Cooking Time : 12 minutes

Servings : 4

Difficulty Level : Easy

Ingredients:

1 cup quinoa

2 cup milk

1 teaspoon vanilla extract

1 teaspoon honey

2 bananas, sliced

¼ teaspoon ground cinnamon

Directions:

1. Pour milk in the saucepan and add quinoa. Close the lid and cook it over the medium heat for 12

minutes or until quinoa will absorb all liquid. Then chill the quinoa for 10-15 minutes and place

in the serving mason jars.

2. Add honey, vanilla extract, and ground cinnamon. Stir well. Top quinoa with banana and stirs it

before serving.

Nutrition (for 100g): 279 Calories 3g Fat 6g Carbohydrates 7g Protein 581mg Sodium

Egg Casserole with Paprika

Preparation Time : 10 minutes

Cooking Time : 28 minutes

Servings : 4

Difficulty Level : Average

Ingredients:

2 eggs, beaten

1 red bell pepper, chopped

1 chili pepper, chopped

½ red onion, diced

1 teaspoon canola oil

½ teaspoon salt

1 teaspoon paprika1 tablespoon fresh cilantro, chopped

1 garlic clove, diced

1 teaspoon butter, softened

¼ teaspoon chili flakes

Directions:

1. Brush the casserole mold with canola oil and pour beaten

eggs inside. After this, toss the butter

in the skillet and melt it over the medium heat. Add chili pepper and red bell pepper.

2. After this, add red onion and cook the vegetables for 7-8 minutes over the medium heat. Stir

them from time to time. Transfer the vegetables in the casserole mold.

3. Add salt, paprika, cilantro, diced garlic, and chili flakes. Stir mildly with the help of a spatula to

get a homogenous mixture. Bake the casserole for 20 minutes at 355F in the oven. Then chill the

meal well and cut into servings. Transfer the casserole in the serving plates with the help of the

spatula.

Nutrition (for 100g): 68 Calories 5g Fat 1g Carbohydrates 4g Protein 882mg Sodium

Cauliflower Fritters

Preparation Time : 10 minutes

Cooking Time : 10 minutes

Servings : 2

Difficulty Level : Easy

Ingredients :

1 cup cauliflower, shredded

1 egg, beaten

1 tablespoon wheat flour, whole grain

1 oz Parmesan, grated

½ teaspoon ground black pepper

1 tablespoon canola oil

Directions:

1. In the mixing bowl mix up together shredded cauliflower and egg. Add wheat flour, grated

Parmesan, and ground black pepper. Stir the mixture with the help of the fork until it is

homogenous and smooth.

2. Pour canola oil in the skillet and bring it to boil. Make the fritters from the cauliflower mixture

with the help of the fingertips or use spoon and transfer in the hot oil. Roast the fritters for 4 minutes from each side over the medium-low heat.

Nutrition (for 100g): 167 Calories 3g Fat 5g Carbohydrates 8g Protein 705mg Sodium

Creamy Oatmeal with Figs

Preparation Time : 10 minutes

Cooking Time : 20 minutes

Servings : 5

Difficulty Level : Easy

Ingredients:

2 cups oatmeal

1 ½ cup milk

1 tablespoon butter

3 figs, chopped

1 tablespoon honey

Directions:

1. Pour milk in the saucepan. Add oatmeal and close the lid. Cook the oatmeal for 15 minutes over

the medium-low heat. Then add chopped figs and honey.

2. Add butter and mix up the oatmeal well. Cook it for 5 minutes more. Close the lid and let the

cooked breakfast rest for 10 minutes before serving.

Nutrition (for 100g): 222 Calories 6g Fat 4g Carbohydrates 1g Protein 822mg Sodium

Baked Oatmeal with Cinnamon

Preparation Time : 10 minutes

Cooking Time : 25 minutes

Servings : 4

Difficulty Level : Easy

Ingredients:

1 cup oatmeal

1/3 cup milk

1 pear, chopped

1 teaspoon vanilla extract

1 tablespoon Splenda

1 teaspoon butter

½ teaspoon ground cinnamon

1 egg, beaten

Directions:

1. In the big bowl mix up together oatmeal, milk, egg, vanilla extract, Splenda, and ground

cinnamon. Melt butter and add it in the oatmeal mixture. Then add chopped pear and stir it well.

2. Transfer the oatmeal mixture in the casserole mold and flatten gently. Cover it with the foil and

secure edges. Bake the oatmeal for 25 minutes at 350F.

Nutrition (for 100g): 151 Calories 9g Fat 3g Carbohydrates 9g Protein 753mg Sodium

Almond Chia Porridge

Preparation Time : 10 minutes

Cooking Time : 30 minutes

Servings : 4

Difficulty Level : Easy

Ingredients:

3 cups organic almond milk

1/3 cup chia seeds, dried

1 teaspoon vanilla extract

1 tablespoon honey

¼ teaspoon ground cardamom

Directions:

1. Pour almond milk in the saucepan and bring it to boil. Then chill the almond milk to the room

temperature (or appx. For 10-15 minutes). Add vanilla extract, honey, and ground cardamom.

Stir well. After this, add chia seeds and stir again. Close the lid and let chia seeds soak the liquid

for 20-25 minutes. Transfer the cooked porridge into the serving ramekins.

Nutrition (for 100g): 150 Calories 3g Fat 1g Carbohydrates 7g Protein 836mg Sodium

Cocoa Oatmeal

Preparation Time : 10 minutes

Cooking Time : 15 minutes

Servings : 2

Difficulty Level : Easy

Ingredients:

1 ½ cup oatmeal

1 tablespoon cocoa powder

½ cup heavy cream

¼ cup of water

1 teaspoon vanilla extract

1 tablespoon butter

2 tablespoons Splenda

Directions :

1. Mix up together oatmeal with cocoa powder and Splenda. Transfer the mixture in the saucepan.

Add vanilla extract, water, and heavy cream. Stir it gently with the help of the spatula.

2. Close the lid and cook it for 10-15 minutes over the medium-low heat. Remove the cooked cocoa

oatmeal from the heat and add butter. Stir it well.Nutrition (for 100g): 230 Calories 6g Fat 5g Carbohydrates 6g Protein 691mg Sodium

Cinnamon Roll Oats

Preparation Time : 7 minutes

Cooking Time : 10 minutes

Servings : 4

Difficulty Level : Easy

Ingredients:

½ cup rolled oats

1 cup milk

1 teaspoon vanilla extract

1 teaspoon ground cinnamon

2 teaspoon honey

2 tablespoons Plain yogurt

1 teaspoon butter

Directions:

1. Transfer milk in the saucepan and bring it to boil. Add rolled oats and stir well. Close the lid and

simmer the oats for 5 minutes over the medium heat. The

cooked oats will absorb all milk.

2. Then add butter and stir the oats well. In the separated bowl, whisk together Plain yogurt with

honey, cinnamon, and vanilla extract. Transfer the cooked oats in the serving bowls. Top the oats

with the yogurt mixture in the shape of the wheel.

Nutrition (for 100g): 243 Calories 2g Fat 1g Carbohydrates 3g Protein 697mg Sodium

Pumpkin Oatmeal with Spices

Preparation Time : 10 minutes

Cooking Time : 13 minutes

Servings : 6

Difficulty Level : Easy

Ingredients :

2 cups oatmeal

1 cup of coconut milk

1 cup milk

1 teaspoon Pumpkin pie spices

2 tablespoons pumpkin puree

1 tablespoon Honey

½ teaspoon butter

Directions:

1. Pour coconut milk and milk in the saucepan. Add butter and bring the liquid to boil. Add oatmeal,

stir well with the help of a spoon and close the lid.

2. Simmer the oatmeal for 7 minutes over the medium heat. Meanwhile, mix up together honey,

pumpkin pie spices, and pumpkin puree. When the oatmeal is cooked, add pumpkin puree

mixture and stir well. Transfer the cooked breakfast in the serving plates.

3. Nutrition (for 100g): 232 Calories 5g Fat 8g Carbohydrates 9g Protein 708mg Sodium

Stewed Cinnamon Apples with Dates
Preparation Time : 15 minutes

Cooking Time : 10 minutes

Servings : 6

Difficulty Level : Easy

Ingredients:

4 large Pink Lady apples

½ cup water

¼ cup chopped pitted dates

1 teaspoon ground cinnamon

¼ teaspoon vanilla extract

1 teaspoon unsalted butterDirections:

1. Place apples, water, dates, and cinnamon in the Instant Pot®. Close, let steam release, press the

Manual button, and set the timer to 3 minutes.

2. When the alarm beeps, quick-release the pressure until the float valve sets. Click the Cancel

button and open lid. Stir in vanilla and butter. Serve hot or chilled.

Nutrition (for 100g): 111 Calories 2g Fat 6g Carbohydrates 1g Protein 411mg Sodium

Spiced Poached Pears

Preparation Time : 10 minutes

Cooking Time : 15 minutes

Servings : 4

Difficulty Level : Easy

Ingredients:

2 cups water

2 cups red wine

¼ cup honey

4 whole cloves

2 cinnamon sticks

1-star anise

1 teaspoon vanilla bean paste

4 Bartlett pears, peeled

Directions:

1. Place all elements in the Instant Pot® and mix. Cover, set steam release to Sealing, press the

Manual Instant Pot®. Stir to couple. Close lid, let steam release to Seal click the Manual button,

and alarm to 3 minutes.

2. When the timer beeps, swiftly-release the pressure until the float valve drops. Select the Cancel

and open. Take out pears to a plate and allow to cool for 5 minutes. Serve warm.

Nutrition (for 100g): 194 Calories 5g Fat 4g Carbohydrates

1g Protein 366mg Sodium

Cranberry Applesauce

Preparation Time : 10 minutes

Cooking Time : 20 minutes

Servings : 8

Difficulty Level : Easy

Ingredients:

1 cup whole cranberries

4 medium tart apples, peeled, cored, and grated

4 medium sweet apples, peeled, cored, and grated

1½ tablespoons grated orange zest

¼ cup orange juice

¼ cup dark brown sugar

¼ cup granulated sugar

1 tablespoon unsalted butter

2 teaspoons ground cinnamon

½ teaspoon ground cloves

¼ teaspoon ground black pepper

1/8 teaspoon salt

1 tablespoon lemon juice

Directions:

1. Incorporate all ingredients in the Instant Pot®. Seal then, set the Manual button, and time to 5

minutes. When the timer beeps, let pressure release naturally, about 25 minutes. Open the lid.

Lightly mash fruit with a fork. Stir well. Serve warm or cold.

Nutrition (for 100g): 136 Calories 4g Fat 3g Carbohydrates

9g Protein 299mg Sodium

Blueberry Compote

Preparation Time : 10 minutes

Cooking Time : 0 minutesServings : 8

Difficulty Level : Average

Ingredients:

1 (16-ounce) bag frozen blueberries, thawed

¼ cup sugar

1 tablespoon lemon juice

2 tablespoons cornstarch

2 tablespoons water

¼ teaspoon vanilla extract

¼ teaspoon grated lemon zest

Directions:

1. Add blueberries, sugar, and lemon juice to the Instant Pot®. Cover and press the Manual button,

and adjust time to 1 minute.

2. When the timer beeps, sharply-release the pressure until the float valve falls. Press the Cancel

button and open it.

3. Press the Sauté button. Combine cornstarch and water. Stir into blueberry mixture and cook

until mixture comes to a boil and thickens, about 3–4 minutes. Press the Cancel button and stir

in vanilla and lemon zest. Serve immediately or refrigerate until ready to serve.

Nutrition (for 100g): 57 Calories 2g Fat 14g Carbohydrates 7g Protein 348mg Sodium

Dried Fruit Compote

Preparation Time : 5 minutes

Cooking Time : 20 minutes

Servings : 6

Difficulty Level : Average

Ingredients:

8 ounces dried apricots, quartered

8 ounces dried peaches, quartered

1 cup golden raisins

1½ cups orange juice

1 cinnamon stick

4 whole cloves

Directions:

1. Stir to merge. Close, select the Manual button, and adjust the time to 3 minutes. When the timer

beeps, let pressure release naturally, about 20 minutes. Press the Cancel button and open lid.

2. Remove and discard cinnamon stick and cloves. Press the Sauté button and simmer for 5–6

minutes. Serve warm then cover and refrigerate for up to a week.

Nutrition (for 100g): 258 Calories 5g Fat 8g Carbohydrates 4g Protein 277mg Sodium

Chocolate Rice Pudding

Preparation Time : 10 minutes

Cooking Time : 20 minutes

Servings : 6

Difficulty Level : Easy

Ingredients:

2 cups almond milk

1 cup long-grain brown rice

2 tablespoons Dutch-processed cocoa powder

¼ cup maple syrup

1 teaspoon vanilla extract

½ cup chopped dark chocolate

Directions:

1. Place almond milk, rice, cocoa, maple syrup, and vanilla in the Instant Pot®. Close then select

the Manual button, and set time to 20 minutes. When the

timer beeps, let pressure release

naturally for 15 minutes, then quick-release the remaining pressure. Press the Cancel button andopen lid. Serve warm, sprinkled with chocolate.

Nutrition (for 100g): 271 Calories 8g Fat 4g Carbohydrates 3g Protein 360mg Sodium

Fruit Compote

Preparation Time : 10 minutes

Cooking Time : 15 minutes

Servings : 6

Difficulty Level : Average

Ingredients:

1 cup apple juice

1 cup dry white wine

2 tablespoons honey

1 cinnamon stick

¼ teaspoon ground nutmeg

1 tablespoon grated lemon zest

1½ tablespoons grated orange zest

3 large apples, peeled, cored, and chopped

3 large pears, peeled, cored, and chopped

½ cup dried cherries

Directions:

1. Situate all ingredients in the Instant Pot® and stir well. Close and select the Manual button, and

allow to sit for 1 minute. When the timer beeps, rapidly-release the pressure until the float valve

hit the bottom. Click the Cancel then open lid.

2. Use a slotted spoon to transfer fruit to a serving bowl. Remove and discard cinnamon stick. Press

the Sauté button and bring juice in the pot to a boil. Cook, stirring constantly, until reduced to a

syrup that will coat the back of a spoon, about 10 minutes.

3. Stir syrup into fruit mixture. Once cool slightly, then wrap with plastic and chill overnight.

Nutrition (for 100g): 211 Calories 1g Fat 4g Carbohydrates

2g Protein 208mg Sodium

Stuffed Apples

Preparation Time : 10 minutes

Cooking Time : 15 minutes

Servings : 6

Difficulty Level : Difficult

Ingredients:

½ cup apple juice

¼ cup golden raisins

¼ cup chopped toasted walnuts

2 tablespoons sugar

½ teaspoon grated orange zest

½ teaspoon ground cinnamon

4 large cooking apples

4 teaspoons unsalted butter

1 cup water

Directions:

1. Put apple juice in a microwave-safe container; heat for 1 minute on high or until steaming and

hot. Pour over raisins. Soak raisins for 30 minutes. Drain, reserving apple juice. Add nuts, sugar,

orange zest, and cinnamon to raisins and stir to mix.

2. Cut off the top fourth of each apple. Peel the cut portion and chop it, then stir diced apple pieces

into raisin mixture. Hollow out and core apples by cutting to, but not through, the bottoms.

3. Situate each apple on a piece of aluminum foil that is large enough to wrap apple completely. Fill

apple centers with raisin mixture.

4. Top each with 1 teaspoon butter. Cover the foil around each apple, folding the foil over at the top

and then pinching it firmly together.

5. Stir in water to the Instant Pot® and place rack inside. Place apples on the rack. Close lid, set

steam release to Sealing, press the Manual, and alarm to 10 minutes.

6. When the timer beeps, quick-release the pressure until the float valve drops and open the lid.

Carefully lift apples out of the Instant Pot®. Unwrap and transfer to plates. Serve hot, at roomtemperature, or cold.

Nutrition (for 100g): 432 Calories 16g Fat 6g Carbohydrates 3g Protein 361mg Sodium

Cinnamon-Stewed Dried Plums with Greek Yogurt

Preparation Time : 10 minutes

Cooking Time : 15 minutes

Servings : 6

Difficulty Level : Easy

Ingredients:

3 cups dried plums

2 cups water

2 tablespoons sugar

2 cinnamon sticks

3 cups low-fat plain Greek yogurt

Directions:

1. Add dried plums, water, sugar, and cinnamon to the Instant Pot®. Close allow steam release to

Sealing, press the Manual button, and start the time to 3 minutes.

2. Once the timer beeps, quick-release the pressure. Click the Cancel button and open. Remove and

discard cinnamon sticks. Serve warm over Greek yogurt.

Nutrition (for 100g): 301 Calories 2g Fat 3g Carbohydrates 14g Protein 244mg Sodium

Vanilla-Poached Apricots

Preparation Time : 10 minutes

Cooking Time : 20 minutes

Servings : 6

Difficulty Level : Average

Ingredients:

1¼ cups water

¼ cup marsala wine

¼ cup sugar

1 teaspoon vanilla bean paste

8 medium apricots, sliced in half and pitted

Directions:

1. Place all pieces in the Instant Pot® and combine well. Seal tight, click the Manual Instant Pot®.

Stir to combine. Close lid, set steam release to Sealing, press the Manual button, and set second

to 1 minute.

2. When the alarm beeps, quick-release the pressure until the float valve drops. Set the Cancel and

open lid. Let stand for 10 minutes. Carefully remove apricots from poaching liquid with a slotted

spoon. Serve warm or at room temperature.

Nutrition (for 100g): 62 Calories 1g Fat 5g Carbohydrates 2g Protein 311mg Sodium

Creamy Spiced Almond Milk

Preparation Time : 10 minutes

Cooking Time : 15 minutes

Servings : 6

Difficulty Level : Average

Ingredients:

1 cup raw almonds

5 cups filtered water, divided

1 teaspoon vanilla bean paste

½ teaspoon pumpkin pie spice

Directions:

1. Stir in almonds and 1 cup water to the Instant Pot®. Close and select the Manual, and set timeto 1 minute.

2. When the timer alarms, quick-release the pressure until the float valve drops. Click the Cancel

button and open cap. Strain almonds and rinse under cool water. Transfer to a high-powered

blender with remaining 4 cups water. Purée for 2 minutes on high speed.

3. Incorporate mixture into a nut milk bag set over a large bowl. Squeeze bag to extract all liquid.

Stir in vanilla and pumpkin pie spice. Transfer to a Mason jar or sealed jug and refrigerate for 8

hours. Stir or shake gently before serving.

Nutrition (for 100g): 86 Calories 8g Fat 5g Carbohydrates 3g Protein 259mg Sodium

Poached Pears with Greek Yogurt and Pistachio

Preparation Time : 10 minutes

Cooking Time : 15 minutes

Servings : 8

Difficulty Level : Average

Ingredients:

2 cups water

1¾ cups apple cider

¼ cup lemon juice

1 cinnamon stick

1 teaspoon vanilla bean paste

4 large Bartlett pears, peeled

1 cup low-fat plain Greek yogurt

½ cup unsalted roasted pistachio meats

Directions:

1. Add water, apple cider, lemon juice, cinnamon, vanilla, and pears to the Instant Pot®. Close lid,

set steam release, switch the Manual, and set time to 3 minutes.

2. When the timer stops, swift-release the pressure until the float valve drops. Select the Cancel

button and open cap. Take out pears to a plate and allow to cool to room temperature.

3. To serve, carefully slice pears in half with a sharp paring knife and scoop out core with a melon

baller. Lay pear halves on dessert plates or in shallow bowls. Top with yogurt and garnish with

pistachios. Serve immediately.

Nutrition (for 100g): 181 Calories 7g Fat 5g Carbohydrates 7g Protein 253mg Sodium

Peaches Poached in Rose Water

Preparation Time : 10 minutes

Cooking Time : 20 minutes

Servings : 6

Difficulty Level : Average

Ingredients:

1 cup water

1 cup rose water

¼ cup wildflower honey

8 green cardamom pods, lightly crushed

1 teaspoon vanilla bean paste

6 large yellow peaches, pitted and quartered

½ cup chopped unsalted roasted pistachio meats

Directions:

1. Add water, rose water, honey, cardamom, and vanilla to the Instant Pot®. Whisk well, then add

peaches. Close lid, allow to steam release to Seal, press the Manual button, and alarm time to 1

minute.

2. When done, release the pressure until the float valve hits the bottom. Press the Remove and

open it. Allow peaches to stand for 10 minutes. Carefully remove peaches from poaching liquid

with a slotted spoon.

3. Slip skins from peach slices. Arrange slices on a plate and garnish with pistachios. Serve warm

or at room temperature.Nutrition (for 100g): 145 Calories 3g Fat 6g Carbohydrates 2g Protein 281mg Sodium

Brown Betty Apple Dessert

Preparation Time : 10 minutes

Cooking Time : 10 minutes

Servings :

Difficulty Level : Difficult

Ingredients:

2 cups dried bread crumbs

½ cup sugar

1 teaspoon ground cinnamon

3 tablespoons lemon juice

1 tablespoon grated lemon zest

1 cup olive oil, divided

8 medium apples, peeled, cored, and diced

2 cups water

Directions:

1. Combine crumbs, sugar, cinnamon, lemon juice, lemon zest, and ½ cup oil in a medium mixing

bowl. Set aside.

2. In a greased oven-safe dish that will fit in your cooker loosely, add a thin layer of crumbs, then

one diced apple. Continue filling the container with alternating layers of crumbs and apples until

all ingredients are finished. Pour remaining ½ cup oil on top.

3. Pour water to the Instant Pot® and place rack inside. Make a foil sling by folding a long piece of

foil in half lengthwise and lower the uncovered container into the pot using the sling.

4. Seal and press the Manual button, and set time to 10 minutes. When the timer stops, let

pressure release naturally, about 20 minutes. Press the Cancel button and open lid. Using the

sling, remove the baking dish from the pot and let stand for 5 minutes before serving.

Nutrition (for 100g): 422 Calories 27g Fat 4g Carbohydrates 7g Protein 355mg Sodium

CPSIA information can be obtained
at www.ICGtesting.com
Printed in the USA
BVHW040321120521
607043BV00001B/248